# ESSENTIALS OF
# DIABETES MELLITUS
# AND
# ITS TREATMENT BY
# HOMOEOPATHY

# ESSENTIALS OF
# DIABETES MELLITUS
### AND
### ITS TREATMENT BY
# HOMOEOPATHY

**Dr. SHAHRUKH KEKI R. PAVRI**
B.H.M.S.

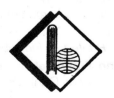

## B. JAIN PUBLISHERS PVT. LTD.
## NEW DELHI - 110 055

**Price: Rs. 20.00**

First edition, 1992

**Reprint edition 1995, 2001**

Published by

**KULDEEP JAIN**

*for*

**B. Jain Publishers (P) Ltd.**

1921, Chuna Mandi, St. 10th, Paharganj,
New Delhi-110 055  3·50
Ph: 3670430, 3670572, 3683200, 3683300
Fax: 011-3610471 & 3683400
Website: www.bjainindia.com, Email: bjain@vsnl.com

*Printed in India by*
**Unisons Techno Financial Consultants (P) Ltd.**
522, FIE, Patpar Ganj, Delhi-110 092

ISBN 81-7021-639-7
*BOOK CODE B-3770*

*This book is dedicated to the memory of my*
GRANDPARENTS.

This book is dedicated to the memory of my

# TABLE OF CONTENTS

# TABLE OF CONTENTS

# PREFACE

When I started my practice, one of my first patients was a neighbour of mine who was suffering from diabetic neuropathy. It was while treating him that I discovered how poor our literature is with regard to good references on Diabetes and worse was the paucity of references regarding the management of the complications of Diabetes. Besides what little was mentioned was scattered far and wide.

Not having too many patients at that time I had ample free time and I put it to good use reading and putting together all that I could lay my hands on. There are three books dealing with the Homoeopathic management of Diabetes but each leaves a lot to be desired when one is looking for the entire view on Diabetes.

In this volume I have attempted to give everything that is known about Diabetes — the nature of the problem, its cause, its clinical presentation and of course its Homoeopathic treatment. Also included is a chapter on dietetics which gives advice, albeit sketchily, on what to eat, what to avoid and more importantly why to avoid it.

The book is written keeping in mind the requirements of the practising Homoeopath as well as students of Homoeopathy though it is written in simple enough style for even the patient himself to understand.

Though a lot of attention has been paid to the preparation of this work, it is just possible that a few mistakes may have crept in. I here and now apologise for any such error. Any constructive criticism would be gladly accepted.

Bombay, November 1991

# ACKNOWLEDGEMENTS

This book would not have been possible without the guidence I have received from :

**Dr. Farokh J. Master L.C.E.H.**
My Guru in Homoeopathy. From him I have learned that curing the incurable is possible; all it needs is to put in enough hard work.

**Dr. S.S. Deshpande M.D.**
From him I learned how to practise medicine and to treat each patient as an individual and not just another 'case'.

**Dr. Kirpal Singh Bakshi D.M.S.**
He showed me that mastering Homoeopathic Materia-Medica is not as daunting a task as it seems.

I would further like to thank :

My parents - without whom this book just was not possible.

Mr. Pervez M. Bhada,
Dr. Jeroo P. Bhada,
Dr. R.D. Edibam,
Dr. M.P. Arya
Dr. D.B. Gaware
Dr. C.S. Sharma
Dr. M.A. Yaveri
Dr. M.V. Botre
Dr. S.D. Petigara
Dr. V.N. Nagpal

Dr. M.P. Vora
Dr. F.M. Najmudeen
Dr. D.A. Pooran
Dr. N.N. Bamji
Dr. N.J. Panthaky
Dr. S. Lulla
Dr. Z.P. Marolia
Dr. K.E. Kodia
Dr. S. Kanakia
Miss D.B. Minbattiwala

# INTRODUCTION

Diabetes Mellitus is a condition of impaired carbohydrate utilisation (clinically characterised by Hyperglycaemia) caused by an absolute or relative deficiency of or resistance to INSULIN. Lack of insulin, whether relative or absolute, affects the metabolism of Carbohydrate, Protein, Lipids, Electrolytes and water, with consequences that might be grave. The chronically deranged metabolism is associated with permanent and essentially irreversible functional and structural changes in the cells of the body. These changes are responsible for the development of clinical entities, the 'complications' of Diabetes Mellitus which affect mainly the Cardio-vascular system, the Eyes, the Kidneys and the Nervous system.

The disease had been recognised since antiquity, and is of particular importance because of its prevalence. The name is derived from the Greek; Diabetes means siphon, signifying the copious amounts of urine passed by the sufferer; Mellitus (= Honey) derives from the sweet taste of the urine due to the glycosuria resulting from elevated levels of blood glucose.

Diabetes Mellitus is a disorder which often does not hurt, is not contagious and is not visible. A Diabetic will not be affected in education, professional training, occupation, family life, enjoyment of leisure hours and an almost full life in old age.

Diabetes affects about 3% of the Indian Population.

# 1.
# CLASSIFICATION OF DIABETES MELLITUS.

1.  Insulin Dependent Diabetes Mellitus (IDDM), or Type I diabetes. Also called Juvenile onset diabetes or Ketosis - prone diabetes or Brittle diabetes.

2.  Non Insulin Dependent Diabetes Mellitus (NIDDM), or Type II diabetes, also called Maturity onset or adult onset or non - ketotic diabetes. It can further be classified as :-

    a)  Obese.

    b)  Non - obese

3.  Secondary Diabetes i.e. diabetes caused by :-

    a)  Pancreatic disease - acute and chronic pancreatitis, carcinoma of pancreas, haemochromatosis, pancreatectomy.

    b)  Hormonal influences - excessive or ectopic secretion of insulin antagonist hormones like:

        i)   Somatotrophin or Growth Hormone secreted by the anterior pituitary (Acromegaly)

        ii)  Catecholamines (Phaeochromocytoma)

        iii) Glucocorticoids (Cushing's syndrome)

        iv)  Glucagon (Glucagonoma)

    c)  Drug induced - Thiazide diuretics, Glucocorticoids, Phenytoin are known to produce an altered glucose tolerance test.

d) Associated with specific genetic disorders like Lipodystrophy, Ataxia - telangectasia.

4. Impaired Glucose Tolerance. Formerly called Latent, Chemical, or Subclinical diabetes.

5. Gestational Diabetes. Sometimes glucose intolerance develops with onset of pregnancy.

6. Potential Diabetes. A person with a normal glucose tolerance, but with an increased potential risk of developing diabetes such as -

   i) An identical twin, the other being diabetic.

   ii) A person with both parents diabetic.

   iii) A person with one parent diabetic and the other parent having a first degree relative who is diabetic.

   iv) A woman who has given birth to a live or stillborn child weighing 4 kilograms or more.

2

# 2.
# AETIOLOGY OF DIABETES MELLITUS

The disease appears to be determined by several different factors rather than by a single cause. A number of these factors are now recognised.

**I.** ***Inadequate Insulin Production.***

    a.     Pancreatic disease : like acute and chronic pancreatitis, carcinoma of pancreas, pancreatectomy.

    b.     Genetic factors - Diabetes is recognised as having a familial tendency. The increased risk of developing IDDM is HLA linked and is primarily associated with the D locus. NIDDM is not HLA linked. Studies have shown that genetic factors are more important in the development of this type of diabetes than in IDDM, but there is little information about what is inherited.

           The insulin gene, situated on the short arm of chromosome 11, has been investigated as a possible genetic marker for NIDDM. Three alleles have been demonstrated - UU, LL and UL. UU seems to affect Blood Glucose homoeostasis and may confer susceptibility to NIDDM.

    c.     Auto-immunity - Circulating antibodies to islet cells can be demonstrated in a vast majority of cases with juvenile onset diabetes. Similar antibodies are also found in a few patients with the maturity onset form of diabetes, most of whom later become insulin dependent. This suggests that in some sub-jects at least, the disease is induced by an auto-immune process.

Circulating antibodies to Thyroid, Gastric mucosa, and the Adrenals are far more common in patients of IDDM than in normal persons. A vast majority of patients with IDDM have demonstrable titres of plasma islet cell antibodies.

d. Viruses - Several pieces of evidence point to the role of viruses in the aetiology of IDDM.

— A clinical history of preceding viral ill-ness, particularly Coxsackie - B and Mumps has been reported before the onset of IDDM.

— Increased viral titres including Coxsackie - B virus, have been reported in IDDM patients at or around the time of onset of the disease.

— Certain diabetogenic viruses (Coxsack-ievirus B. Encephalomyocarditis M. and Rheovirus) can cause diabetes when innoculated into rodents.

— Diabetogenic viruses can also directly infect Beta-cells in culture causing cell lysis and cell death.

— Autopsy reports of patients dying within a few months of onset of IDDM show an 'insulitis' consisting of round cell infiltra-tion of cell tissue.

e. Drugs - Certain drugs such as the Thiazide diuretics, Phloridzin, Alloxan and others can induce diabetes; the diabetogenic effect of Thiazide diuretics is reversible, that of Alloxan is not.

4

## II.  *Insulin  Antagonism.*

a.   Endocrine - Diabetes Mellitus may develop when hormones with insulin antagonist properties are produced in excess.

   i.    Somatotrophin or Growth hormone - as in Acromegaly.

   ii.   Glucocorticoids - as in Cushing's syndrome or in patients requiring treatment with high doses of corticosteriods.

   iii)  Catecholamines - as in Phaeochromocytoma.

   iv)   Glucagon - as in Glucagonoma.

b.   Obesity  - The prevalence of Diabetes Mellitus is approximately three times higher in overweight than in non-overweight persons. Diabetes Mellitus develops only with the appropriate genetic legacy, but obesity, by enhancing insulin resistance, increases the demand on the pancreatic islets and tends to unmask and exacerbate the underlying propensity to Diabetes.

c.   Pregnancy - Diabetes may present during pregnancy or established diabetes may become worse. Furthermore there is an increased incidence of the condition in multiparous women as compared with those who had no children. Human Placental Lactogen, synthetized by the placenta, is an insulin antagonist similar in many respects to Growth  hormone.

d.   Others - Several other insulin antagonists have been described. The most important are fatty acids; their importance in the aetiology of Diabetes is not well understood.

5

# 3.
# PATHOLOGY

In IDDM the pancreatic islet tissue shows degeneration, in which the Beta-cells are destroyed, leaving only Alpha cells and other undifferentiated cells. The existing Beta cells show evidence of increased activity with enlarged nuclei and degranulation of the cytoplasm. The microscopic appearance of the Pancreas is consistent with the low levels of plasma insulin found in these patients.

In NIDDM the impaired peripheral utilisation of glucose is out of proportion to the reduction in the mass of islet tissue. The Beta cells show failure to develop cytological signs of overactivity despite the chronic hyperglycemia and reduction in number of Beta cells. This suggests that the Beta cells are insensitive to the stimulus of hyperglycemia.

The pathological changes underlying the 'complications' of diabetes will be discussed later alongwith the complications.

## CHEMICAL PATHOLOGY.

The basic metabolic fault is the deficiency of insulin which results in hyperglycemia. The deficiency is absolute in IDDM but is only relative in NIDDM. Basically this produces a situation of glucose lack and increased Gluconeogenesis and Lipolysis follow as compensatory reaction under the influence of hormones such as Growth hormone, Glucagon and Glucocorticoids. Thus the hyperglycemia of Diabetes arises from two basic mechanisms, namely a reduced rate of glucose pick-up from the blood by the peripheral tissues and an increased rate of release of glucose from the liver into the circulation.

Blood glucose concentration in excess of the capacity of the renal tubules to reabsorb it, results in glycosuria i.e. passing glucose in the urine. In most people this occurs when the blood glucose level reaches or surpasses 180 mg/100 ml (10 mmol/litre).Glucose increases the osrnolality of the glomerular filtrate and thus blocks the tubular reabsorption of water. This greatly increases the volume of urine resulting in polyuria and nocturia. The ensuing severe loss of water and solutes is sought to be compensated by Thirst and Polydipsia.

Poor carbohydrate utilisation results in a sense of Fatigue. The body compensates by initiating two mechanisms to provide alternative metabolic fuel. Both these mechanisms ultimately lead to wasting (loss of body tissue) which occurs in spite of normal or even increased nutritional intake. These compensatory mechanisms are -

i.   Increased  Glycogenolysis  and  Gluconeogenesis.

The catabolism of glycogen and protein causes the release of glucose, water and electrolytes from the cells; this leads to increased urinary excretion of Potassium, Magnesium and Phosphorus.

ii.  Increased  lipolysis.

There is an increase in free fatty acids in the plasma. The extent of lypolysis is proportional to the severity of insulin deficiency. In gross insulin deficiency, the normal response of plasma free fatty acids to feeding (drop in lipolysis and thus a drop in free fatty acids) may be lost and plasma free fatty levels may persist at high values.

The liver breaks down fatty acids within its mito-chondria in eight steps, each of which yields one molecule of acetyl co-enzyme A. Normally, most of these molecules are condensed with oxaloacetic acid, but in severe diabetes, more is formed than can enter the Citric acid cycle. The majority of this is reduced to beta-hydroxy-butyric acid, while some is decarboxylated to acetone. This acetone (a ketone) when formed in small amounts is usually utilised as metabolic fuel by oxidation. Thus, when hepatic pro-duction of ketone exceeds the rate of utilisation by the peripheral tissues, the plasma levels rise.

Ketones are strong acids which dissociate easily and release Hydrogen ions into the body fluids. They also increase the osmolality of plasma and lead to the withdrawal of water from the cell. This state of affairs where the ketones and Hydrogen ions in the plasma are raised is called Ketoacidosis.

# 4.
# CLINICAL PRESENTATION

Diabetes is a widely-spread disease and may present in one of several ways.

1.  A large percentage of sufferers present with complaints of some or all of the classical symptoms of diabetes. These are —

    Polydipsia
    Polyuria
    Polyphagia
    Nocturia
    Loss of weight
    Fatigue
    Pruritus Vulvae
    Balanitis or Balanoposthitis
    Impotence
    Changes in refractive error of the eyes.

2.  The patient may be discovered to have Diabetes after routine medical check-up for a variety of reasons. The clinical syndrome may be absent or very few mild symptoms may be present which the patient may not even have noticed.

3.  Diabetes may present as a full-blown Ketoacidosis. This is more likely with IDDM and is an acute medical emergency. Intensive care and insulin alongwith Homoeopathic remedies forms the mainstay of successful treatment.

4. Patients may present with features of the complications of Diabetes; these complications being—
   Diabetic Neuropathy
   Diabetic Vasculopathy
   Diabetic Nephropathy
   Diabetic Occular Disturbances
   Dermatological Complications of Diabetes.

# 5.
# DIAGNOSTIC CRITERIA

The diagnosis of Diabetes Mellitus can be made on the basis of the clinical picture which consists of some or all of the following —-

Polyuria
Polyphagia
Polydipsia
Nocturia
Loss of weight
Pruritus Vulvae
Impotence
Balanitis or Balanoposthitis

The diagnosis must be confirmed by the results of the following laboratory investigations.

Blood Glucose Level  -  Fasting
                      -  Post Prandial
                      -  Glucose Tolerance Test.

Plasma Acetone Level
Urine Sugar
Urine Acetone
Glycosylated Haemoglobin (Haemoglobin A1)
Serum Lipoproteins

**Blood Glucose levels.**

This test is done on venous blood, taking an over-night fasting sample and another sample two hours after a meal. An isolated increased result is to be treated with caution and the test should be repeated after a few days with the patient refraining (if possible) from taking any medication for atleast two or three days prior to the test before labelling the patient as diabetic.

The normal values of Blood glucose are —-

Blood Glucose - Fasting   70 - 100 mg/100 ml
Blood Glucose - Two hours Post prandial       100
140 mg/100 ml

The blood glucose levels are raised in :
    Diabetes Mellitus
    Hemochromatosis
    Cushing's syndrome
    Acromegaly and Gigantism
Injection of Adrenalin
Phaeochromocytoma
Stress (e.g. shock, burns, emotions)
Acute and chronic pancreatitis
Wernicke's encephalopathy (vitamin B1 deficiency)
    Subarachnoid haemorrhage
    Administration of ACTH

**Glucose Tolerance Test. (GTT)**

The glucose tolerance test is a series of blood glucose estimations after a standard glucose load which may be either oral or intravenous. Oral GTT is more useful for diagnosis of Diabetes Mellitus and pancreatic cell hyperactivity. Intravenous GTT is useful to clarify or rule out the influence of absorption factors in the curve. The oral glucose load is standardised at 75 gms. while the intravenous load is calculated as 20% glucose (0.5 gm/kg body weight) intravenously over 30 minutes.

The procedure for the GTT is to collect blood after 10 - 12 hours fasting, then the appropriate glucose load is given and further samples of blood are collected at 1, 2 and 3 hour intervals. The values are plotted on a graph, the glucose tolerance 'curve'.

The normal values are —

| | |
|---|---|
| Fasting | upto 90 mg/100 ml. |
| 60 minutes after 75 gms. oral glucose | upto 160 mg/100 ml. |
| 120 minutes after glucose | upto140 mg/100 ml. |
| 150 minutes after glucose | upto100 mg/100 ml. |

For standardised results, an appropriate prior diet of atleast 250 gm of carbohydrate daily should be prescribed; the patient must abstain from alcohol for 3 days before the test. The patient should be fasting for 10 - 12 hours before the test, with no smoking or drinking of coffee. The test should be postponed if the subject has fever or shows other signs of an infection.

In Diabetes Mellitus the tolerance is decreased. The curve shows an excessive peak (due to decreased utilisation) with a slow fall to fasting level. A similar curve is seen in Hyperlipidemia types III, IV and V; in Haemochromatosis; steroid effect (Cushing's disease, administration of steroids or ACTH) and in CNS lesions.

Elevated fasting blood sugar may be normal in mild diabetes; therefore, it is inadequate for case finding. Elevated 2 hour post-prandial blood sugar alone is superior to fasting blood sugar alone for routine screening for diabetes.

Glucose tolerance test (GTT) is most useful for detecting latent or incipient diabetes. In case the GTT is within normal limits but diabetes mellitus is clinically suspected, the GTT should be repeated. A cortisone challenge increases the sensitivity of the test. A diabetic type of GTT curve may be seen if the patient has not had an adequate intake of carbohydrate and calories.

## Urine sugar

The test for presence of 'sugar' in urine is routinely done using Benedict's reagent. In a test-tube 8 drops of urine are mixed with 5 ml. of Benedict's reagent; this mixture is then gently heated. The result is then read from the color of the sediment which settles at the bottom of the test-tube. The significance of the color change is as given below.

| Colour of sediment | Urine sugar |
|---|---|
| Blue | 0 |
| Green | + |
| Yellow | ++ |
| Orange | +++ |
| Red | ++++ |

The drawback of this method is that any reducing substance can give a positive Benedict's test. A positive Benedict's test is obtained in the following conditions.

### i. Glycosuria

  a. Hyperglycemia
   — Endocrine e.g. Diabetes mellitus, pituitary and adrenal disease.
   — Non endocrine e.g. CNS disease.

— Due to hormone administration e.g. ACTH, corticosteroids.

b. Renal tubular origin
   — Renal diabetes
   — Toxic renal tubular disease
   — Inflammatory renal disease e.g. acute glomerulonephritis.

c. Idiopathic

## ii. *Melituria*

a. Hereditary (due to fructose, galactose, pentose, lactose)

b. Neonatal (e.g. sepsis, gastroenteritis)

c. Lactosuria during lactation.

## iii. *Non-sugar reducing substances (e.g. salicylates, ascorbic acid, glucuronic acid)*

## Plasma acetone

Though acetone is a normal component of plasma, it is present in concentrations so low that it is not detected by routine biochemistry. The normal range is 0.3 - 2.0 mg/100ml. An increased level of plasma ketones will result in their excretion in the urine.

## Urinary Ketones.

The ketones that appear in urine are — acetone, beta-hydroxy-butyric acid and acetoacetic acid. Ketonuria occurs in the following conditions.

a. Metabolic
   i. Diabetes Mellitus
   ii. Renal glycosuria

iii. Glycogen storage disease
b. Dietary
    i. High-fat diet
    ii. Starvation
c. Elevated metabolic requirements
    i. Fever
    ii. Thyrotoxicosis
    iii. Pregnancy and lactation

## Glycosylated Haemoglobin (Haemoglobin A1)

Chromatographic fractionation of haemoglobin from a normal person shows a major component HbA and several smaller faster-moving components collectively referred to as HbAI. The transition from HbA to HbAI is brought about by the addition of a glucose group to the terminal amino acid of the beta chain. This reaction is non-enzymatic and post-synthetic (i.e. the glucose group is added on after the haemoglobin molecule has been synthesized, integrated into the RBC and the RBC has been released into the circulation). The rate of synthesis of HbAI is a function of the blood glucose concentration. The glucose linkage is fairly stable and thus HbAI accumulates throughout the life-span of the RBC (about 120 days) and its concentration reflects the average blood glucose concentration over the past three months. Thus the concentration of HbAI is a marker for the quality of control of Diabetes in the preceding few months. The normal value of HbAI concentration is taken as upto 8%.

## Serum Lipoproteins

Diabetes is known to affect the metabolism of lipids. Hyperlipoproteinemias are classified on the

16

basis of which class of lipoprotein is elevated. Diabetes is most commonly associated with Type 4 and less commonly with Type 5 Hyperlipoproteinemia.

A Diabetic Hyperlipoproteinemia shows elevated levels of chylomicrons and VLDL (very low density lipoproteins). The mechanism of hyperlipoproteinemia in Diabetes is the increased secretion of VLDL coupled with a decreased catabolism of VLDL and/ or chylomicrons due to diminished lipoprotein lipase activity. Insulin deficiency and/or resistance is associated with all class s of hyperlipoproteinemia to a greater or smaller extent.

The normal values of serum lipoproteins varies with the laboratory and therefore, the reference values given by the laboratory should be considered.

17

# 6.
# COMPLICATIONS OF DIABETES MELLITUS

Diabetes Mellitus is a chronic disease and ultimately leads to the establishment of certain well-defined clinical entities which are referred to as the 'complications' of diabetes.

## DIABETIC KETOACIDOSIS

This is caused by a failure on the part of the patient to appreciate the symptoms (and the importance of these symptoms) of poor control of diabetes. There is depletion of water and electrolytes. The water is drawn in equal amounts from the intracellular and the extracellular compartments. The mechanism of water and electrolyte depletion is as follows — the raised level of blood glucose increases the osmolality of the glomerular filtrate and hence blocks water reabsorption by the tubules. This increases the urine output and results in the loss of both Sodium and Potassium. The serum electrolyte levels may not be significantly altered due to a disproportionate loss of water. This loss of water and electrolytes results in haemoconcentration, fall in plasma volume and hypotension with associated renal ischemia and oliguria.

Furthermore, due to the decreased peripheral utilisation of ketones (which are strong acids) in catabolism, a state of Ketoacidosis supervenes. The rise in Hydrogen ion concentration (i.e. fall in pH) and increase in $Pco_2$ in arterial blood stimulate pulmonary

18

ventilation so that clinically hyperpnoea (air hunger or acidotic respiration) is observed.

An acute infection or negligence with respect to treatment or dietary control can precipitate severe ketoacidosis. This applies to even those who are mild diabetics.

The SYMPTOMS of Diabetic Ketoacidosis (DKA) are - intense thirst, polyuria, constipation, alteration in vision, cramps, abdominal pain, vomiting, drowsiness and fatigue.

The SIGNS of DKA are - dry tongue, sunken eyes, acidotic respiration, weak rapid pulse, hypotension, smell of acetone on the breath, and an altered state of consciousness, may be even coma. The coma associated with DKA must not be confused with that due to hypoglycemia; the salient differences are given on the following page.

## Coma due to Ketoacidosis

Preceded by an acute infection, digestive irregularity, inadequate or no insulin, stopping accustomed exercise.

Insidious onset with preceding ill-health for several days.

Skin and tongue are dry i.e. dehydration is present.

Patient is hypotensive with weak pulse.

Air hunger (acidotic respiration)

Reflexes may be diminished or unchanged. Plantar response is extensor

Symptoms of hyperglycemia viz.,
polyuria
polydipsia
thirst

abdominal pain with or without vomiting.

Biochemical profile
  hyperglycemia
  glycosuria present
  ketonuria present
  plasma bicarbonates decreased
  pH is decreased.

## *Coma due to Hypoglycaemia.*

Preceded by missed meals, excess of insulin, un-accustomed physical exertion.
Sudden, rapid onset usually can be traced to last insulin dose.
Skin and tongue are moist i.e. no dehydration.
Patient normotensive or even hypertensive with full pulse.
Normal or shallow respiration.
Reflexes brisk. Plantar response is flexor.
Symptoms of hypoglycaemia viz.,
  weak feeling
  hunger
  sweating
  palpitation, tachycardia
  tremors
  faintness, dizziness
  headache
  diplopia
  mental confusion

Biochemical profile
  hypoglycaemia
  glycosuria absent
  ketonuria absent
  plasma bicarbonates normal
  pH is normal

# DIABETIC NEUROPATHY

Diabetic neuropathy occurs more often in older patients. Poor control of diabetes predisposes to an early onset and increased incidence of diabetic neuropathy. The following are the main categories of neuropathy associated with diabetes.

A. Peripheral neuropathy. It may be -

— Distal, symmetrical, mixed sensory-motor polyneuropathy.

It causes symmetrical, distal paresthesia; glove and stocking sensory loss; distal weakness and loss of ankle jerks.

— Sensory neuropathy

It is distal and symmetrical. It presents with numbness and paresthesiae extending proximally. There is loss of position and vibration sense. Because of the sensory loss, trophic ulcers and Charcot's joints may also be seen.

B. Motor neuropathy
It is in asymmetrical and proximal neuropathy. Also called Diabetic amyotrophy, it presents with asymmetrical wasting of the quadriceps with diminished or absent knee jerks.

C. Mononeuritis multiplex
Several spinal nerves are affected either concurrently or serially. The signs are 'patchy' and asymmetrical.

D. Autonomic neuropathy
This is manifested as
Impotence
Diarrhoea

21

Postural hypotension
Alteration of sweating and micturition
Tachycardia

## DIABETIC VASCULOPATHY

Partial or complete occlusion of blood vessels is the basic pathology here. Large vessels are occluded by atheromatous plaques and smaller vessels (arterioles) by endarteritis. This leads to myocardial infarction, intermittent claudication, diminution or loss of peripheral pulsations and predisposes to gangrene. Many diabetics may suffer from what are termed 'silent' myocardial infarctions i.e. the element of pain is greatly diminished or may even be absent. The incidence of cerebrovascular disease is high in diabetics; the presence of diabetes makes the patient a high risk patient for endarterectomy and besides, the lesions are usually multiple and hence not amenable to surgical treatment.

## DIABETIC NEPHROPATHY

Diabetes predisposes to Pyelonephritis which may be associated with papillary necrosis. Diabetes also results in two kinds of Glomerulosclerosis; one is a diffuse proliferative type and consists of a general thickening of the basement membrane. The other is a nodular variety in which hyaline rounded masses called Kimmelstiel-Wilson bodies are seen, which actually are eosinophilic nodules in the glomerular tuft. Renal vascular changes secondary to atherosclerosis and hypertension may also be seen.

Even well-established diabetic nephropathy may manifest only as mild to moderate proteinuria, though in some cases a full-blown Nephrotic syndrome with

22

consequent renal failure and azotemia may eventually develop.

## DIABETIC OCCULAR DISTURBANCES

The eyes are the most commonly affected organs in long standing diabetes. Fluctuations in plasma osmolality due to changing blood sugar levels cause blurred vision by inducing osmotic fluid and glucose transfer across the capsule of the lens. There is an increased incidence and an earlier onset of cataract in diabetic patients.

The abnormalities comprising diabetic retinopathy are -

— Venous engorgement of retinal vessels
— Capillary microaneurysms
— 'Waxy' exudates
— Retinitis proliferans (new vessel formation)
— Retinal detachment
— Vitreous fibrosis
— Haemorrhage    — 'Blots' (intraretinal)
                 — Preretinal (subhyaloid)
                 — Into the vitreous

Patients with microaneurysms, retinal haemorrhages and exudates are said to have simple or background retinopathy. Those with preretinal haemorrhage, new vessel formation or fibrous proliferation are said to have malignant or proliferative retinopathy.

New vessel formation over the iris (Rubeosis iridis) may lead to blockage of the filtration angle and thus cause glaucoma.

## INCREASED INCIDENCE OF INFECTIONS

Suboptimal control of diabetes is associated with a decreased resistance to infection. The commonest infections are Pulmonary Koch's, Urinary tract infections, Candidiasis and deep mycoses.

## DERMATOLOGICAL COMPLICATIONS OF DIABETES MELLITUS

The commonest of these is insulin induced Lipodystrophy at the site of injection of insulin. Trophic ulcers due to neuropathy or ischemia may progress to gangerene if not energetically treated. Infections like furuncles, carbuncles and candidiasis are common. Many patients show pigmented scars over the shins - the so-called 'shin spots' or diabetic dermopathy. Diabetics may also exhibit various xanthomata secondary to the hyperlipidemia. Necrobiosis lipoidica diabeticorum consists of round or oval, sharply defined, plaque-like lesions on the anterior surface of the lower legs; these plaques are uncommon and tend to ulcerate after the slightest trauma.

# 7.

# GENERAL INSTRUCTIONS FOR PATIENTS OF DIABETES MELLITUS

Patients with diabetes mellitus can lead an almost normal life provided they are careful with diet and diligent with respect to medicines and exercise. The success of treatment is heavily dependent on the patient's co-operation. Though diabetes may be a life long companion, it is not a fate to be resigned to but a skirmish to be fought.

Obesity (considered as 20% more weight than the ideal weight for height and age) can be the forerunner of diabetes. In fact obesity is the first and usually the most easily surmountable obstacle to the successful management of diabetes. Lack of physical exercise is another risk factor for diabetes. This lack of physical exercise leads to obesity and hence sedentary life is a two-tiered risk factor acting both directly and by way of the patient getting overweight. It must be impressed upon the patient that a uniform daily gentle exercise is always to be prefered over sporadic spurts of exhausting exercises or sports. A daily walk wearing good socks and well-fitting shoes is the best exercise one can prescribe for the patient. Of course, age and the presence of complications like atherosclerosis, ischemic heart disease etc. must be kept in mind.

The need to persevere with dietary regulations and exercise schedule even after the levels of blood glucose have normalised must be explained to the patient. Younger patients are more likely to disregard a doctor's advice.

The phenomenon of hypoglycaemia must be brought to the notice of the patient and his relatives. The salient features of hypoglycaemia are — Disorientation, ravenous appetite, outbreaks of sweating, trembling, feeling of weakness, headache, restlessness, formication and palpitation. A known diabetic who looks drunken may actually be suffering from acute hypoglycaemia. The patient may also exhibit certain behavioural changes; some become tearful and depressed, some become aggressive or irritable. Severe hypoglycaemia may lead to convulsive episodes and even loss of consciousness.

The causes of hypoglycaemia are —

i.    Overdosage of insulin or oral hypoglycaemic agents if the patient is concurrently being administered these.

ii.   Delaying or missing a meal.

iii.  Unusually hard work or increased physical activity.

The immediate ingestion of carbohydrates is the best treatment for hypoglycaemia. This can be taken in the form of glucose, cane sugar, a soft drink or sweets. Every diabetic patient must carry with him a little sugar or a few sweets.

The patient and his relatives must also be informed about the other extreme - Hyperglycaemia. Here the blood sugar levels rise to alarmingly high values and can lead to loss of consciousness - Diabetic Coma. Loss of consciousness occurs as a result of dehydration and ketoacidosis. The patient feels lethargic; has great thirst and passes large quantities of urine. Nausea, vomiting and abdominal pains may also occur. The breath smells of acetone and the respiration is rapid and shallow what is called Acidotic respiration.

Diabetic coma is best tackled in a well equipped hospital. Never forget to look for a nidus of infection when the blood sugar rises. The commonest is Pulmonary Tuberculosis.

Every diabetic must carry a card or wear a bracelet which gives his name, address and phone number as well as the name, address and phone number of doctor. It must of course mention prominently that he suffers from Diabetes Mellitus. The patient should be encouraged to regularly monitor his metabolic status using simple dipstick tests. These test strips are easily available; there being differently types for monitoring the level of sugar in urine and blood. Instruct the patient to maintain a diabetics chart and ask him to bring it with him on every visit. Estimation of urine glucose is never a substitute for estimation of blood glucose levels and this must be done on a regular basis.

Instructions pertaining to day-to-day activities must also be given to the patients, these are —

## PERSONAL HYGEINE

The patient must bathe regularly and thoroughly at least once a day. The patient must bathe his feet daily, dry them properly and dust them with talcum powder or swab them with eau de Cologue or spirit. Any skin infections like Ringworm or other mycotic infections must be treated immediately and vigorously. Patient must apply talcum powder frequently to areas of the skin prone to excessive sweating and friction e.g. the groins, axillary folds etc. Good dental hygeine with a regular check-up by a dental surgeon is always beneficial.

## AVOID INJURIES

The smallest of cuts, even abrasions, must be diligently dressed and kept clean. The patient must be instructed to shave carefully; electric shavers are to be preferred as against the use of 'safety' razors.

Cutting finger-and toe-nails must be done after a bath. Nails should never be cut too short; they should be cut in line with the toes. Manicures and pedicures should only be done by experienced personnel. The patient must never walk barefooted.

Strong antiseptics which may burn or irritate the skin, such as tincture iodine, salicylic acid and carbolic acid must be avoided. A one in ten solution of Calendula tincture in water is always the best material for dressing wounds and scratches.

## CARE OF THE FEET

The patient must be advised to avoid tight shoes which may cause corns. Shoes should be broad at the tip so as not to compress the toes. New shoes should only be worn for short periods of time. Warn the patient against cutting corns or applying corncaps. The results may be dangerous.

Regular foot massage, warm socks in winter, avoiding socks with tight elastic bands and a regular walk will go a long way in improving the circulation in the lower extremities.

The patient should aviod wearing underpants that are tight around the thighs and should avoid sitting for long with legs crossed.

## DANGER SIGNALS

The patient must be told to inform the doctor if he notices any of the following :-

— Any injury however minor, wherever on the body it may be.

— Tingling, formication or burning in the feet and/or the hands.

— Numbness or coldness of the feet.

— Cramps in the calves.

— Change of the color of the skin, toes, fingers or nails to dark red or purple.

# 8.
# BASIS OF
# TREATMENT

Here one has to consider two aspects of the treatment of Diabetes Mellitus. Firstly one has the patient who consults you as a Homoeopathic physician for the treatment of Diabetes Mellitus per se. The second class of patients is where one is called in for the management of one or more of the full-blown complications of Diabetes, be it Coma, Gangrene or Multiple Neuritis.

First we shall consider the Principles of management of Daibetes without full-blown complications. The mainstay of the treatment in Diabetes is to follow one of the following regimens -

- Diet alone
- Diet and Homoeopathic medicines
- Diet, Homoeopathic medicines and Insulin.

Regular non-strenuous exercise, the best example of which is walking, is an absolute necessity for the ideal management of Diabetes Mellitus.

Explain in simple words to the patient that he suffers from Diabetes Mellitus, that he is not the first person to suffer from this disease and definitely is not the last. In short, make it very clear that he suffers from a very common disease which in itself may not trouble him but which has the definite potential to give rise to disabling and at times, fatal complications.

The importance of maintaining a good control of the blood sugar is essential as the onset and progress of complications is definitely delayed in patients in whom blood glucose homeostasis is well maintained. Thus it is important to stress upon the necessity of being regular in treatment and of adhering strictly to the regimen of diet and exercise prescribed for the patient.

Diet is considered in detail in a subsequent chapter.

Constitutional remedies must be prescribed on the totality of symptoms and are discussed later in the second part of this work. Auxiliary remedies are to be used as an adjunct to treatment and may be loosely considered as being useful in bringing down the blood sugar levels. It must be remembered that they, in themselves, cannot be expected to CURE and those using only these drugs without recourse to the potentised similimum have but themselves to blame if success eludes them. These drugs are to be used as Tinctures or in low potencies (for e.g. 1X, 2X or 3X).

## The management of complications.

The treatment of complications is to be tackled on the same lines as one would handle any acute condition cropping up in the course of a chronic disease. The principles of treatment are to select a remedy on the SECTOR TOTALITY. This remedy must be administered internally in the potentised form. The choice of the potency must be decided upon the individual merits of the case viz., the susceptibility of the patient and the extent of structural damage, The decision whether to simultaneously administer the constitutional remedy must again be taken on the basis of the signs and symptoms of the case at hand.

## Role of Insulin in Homoeopathic management of Diabetes Mellitus.

The decision regarding the simultaneous admini-stration of Insulin in grave cases or in well-established cases of IDDM is a difficult one to make. The purists would roundly decry the use of insulin, terming it as 'allopathic'. But what one must keep in mind is that Dr. Hahnemann, in sixth edition of ORGANON, has himself advised the use of non-Homoeopathic meas-ures in grave cases where the Vital Energy is too week to attempt to rectify its derangement. Of course, the actual administration and adjustment of the dosage is best left to a person qualified in modern medicine.

# 9.
# MIASMATIC APPROACH

Diabetes Mellitus is classically considered to be of TUBERCULAR origin. All the classical symptoms of Diabetes Mellitus have been mentioned as being Tubercular. The following symptoms have all been grouped under Tubercular miasm or Psuedo-Psora.

— Loss of strength after urinating.

— Copiousness of urine is a tubercular trait.

— The majority of renal difficulties have a Tubercular basis, which can be demonstrated by a careful study of all the latent miasmatic symptoms of the whole person.

— Neuralgic pains are of Tubercular origin.

— Excessive suppuration is a Tubercular trait.

— In abscesses and ulcers of the skin, the Tubercular element is always uppermost.

— Injuries to the skin, especially slight injuries heal readily in the Psoric patients; but it is in the Tubercular individual that we see the abscess, the ulcerative process and the copious formation and elimination of pus, far beyond that necessary in the ordinary healing process.

— Gangrene has a syphilitic or Tubercular taint.

— Perversions of form, shape or size are Tubercular or Syphilitic in origin.

— Hunger with an all-gone sensation in the pit of the stomach is again a Tubercular symptom.

—    The tendency to secondary complications is a Tubercular trait.

Diabetic patients are as a rule strongly Tubercular, with the Tubercular physiology throughout them. If Sycosis is present, these cases are of course more malignant in their nature and more fatal.

Fibrous changes in the kidneys also have the three miasms present although the Tubercular and Sycotic are present in the majority of cases.

IDDM is considered to be due to an auto-immune response and this is classified as an aberrant immune response and hence is a Tubercular trait.

# 10.
# THE HOMOEOPATHIC THERAPEUTICS OF DIABETES MELLITUS

In the following pages I have made an attempt at giving the salient features of the remedies, briefly touching on the most important and relevant symptoms. My only excuse for this is that this is work on THERAPEUTICS and not a MATERIA MEDICA. The choice of the remedy must be made on the totality of symptoms. I have purposely kept the number of general symptoms to a bare (essential) minimum. The prescriber must of course refer to a standard test-book of materia-medica for selecting the similimum on the basis of symptom totality. The materia-medica is, and must always remain, the final court of appeal in remedy selection.

The remedies mentioned in the subsequent pages have been culled from a multitude of sources, the credit for which are all given at the end in the bibliography. The list of remedies is extensive but by no means exhaustive.

I have loosely classified the remedies into two different groups.

The first group consists of a collection of deep-acting constitutional remedies, all well-proved and having a clinically verified symptomatology and some remedies which are not as extensively proved but having an adequate clinical verification in the treatment of Diabetes and the lowering of blood sugar.

This group also includes a set of remedies that have in their symptomatology a disease picture coresponding to one or more of the 'complications' of Diabetes. Here I have paid special attention to Diabetic Pre-Coma, Diabetic Coma and Diabetic Gangrene.

The second group comprises 'rare' remedies where the indications are only a single or very few symptoms and that too these indications are usually common symptoms. These remedies need to be studied further and also need a better proving.

I have purposely not made a mention of any alternative therapy either Hydrotherapy, Naturopathy or the concept of Blood and/or Urine Isotherapy as these are all non-Homoeopathic and hence have no place in a work on the Homoeopathic therapeutics of Diabetes Mellitus.

## LIST OF REMEDIES

### PRINCIPAL REMEDIES

Abroma Augusta
Acetic Acid
Argentum Metallicum
Argentum Nitricum
Arsenicum Album
Boric Acid
Bovista
Bryonia Alba
Carbo Vegetabilis
Carbolic Acid
Causticum
Ceanothus
Cephalandra Indica
Conium Maculatum
Crotalus Horridus

Cuprum Arsenicosum
Cuprum Metallicum
Gymnema Sylvestre
Helleborus Niger
Helonias Dioica
Iodum
Iris Versicolor
Kali Bromatum
Kreosotum
Lachesis
Lactic Acid
Lycopodium Clavatum
Medorrhinum
Morphinum
Moschus

Natrum Muriaticum
Natrum Sulphuricum
Nitric Acid
Nux Vomica
Opium
Phosphoric Acid
Phosphorus
Picric Acid
Plumbum Metallicum
Sanicula Aqua

Secale Cornutum
Sepia
Silicea
Sulphur
Syzygium Jambolanum
Tarentula
Thuja
Uranium Nitricum
Fluoric Acid

## ABROMA AUGUSTA
### (Olat Kambal)

Dry tongue and mouth with intense thirst for large quantity of cold water which does not relieve the dryness. Early, short menses, DYSMENORRHOEA. Voracious appetite, hungry even after a full meal. Profuse urination day and night, with peculiar fishy odor of urine. Glycosuria. Impotence and extreme exhaustion after coitus. General weakness. Constipation. Carbuncles. Sleeplessness. Albuminuria. In general patient is worse in summer, at night in bed.

## ACETIC ACID
### (Glacial Acetic Acid)

Suited to patients who are wasted, debilitated and thirsty. The patient passes large quantities of pale urine and has a tendency to easy and frequest fainting, difficult breathing, and oedema. Gastric fermentation with excessive salivation and burning in the stomach.

## ARGENTUM METALLICUM
### (Silver, the metal)

Tall, thin, irritable persons who desire open air are

37

characteristically affected by this remedy. Diabetics who have chronically swollen ankles. Copious, frequent urination where the urine has a sweetish odour. Violent appetite with emaciation. The patient feels that his limbs have become powerless.

## ARGENTUM NITRICUM
### (Silver Nitrate; $AgNO_3$)

Patients who are dried, withered up and look prematurely old. Neurotics who complain of weakness and trembling. The patients crave sugar but sugar causes diarrhoea. The urine is highly colored and contains albumin and uric acid crystals. Diabetic ulcers with splinter like pains. Impotence. Polyneuritis, numbness of the extremities causing difficulty in walking.

## ARSENIC ALBUM
### (While oxide of arsenic, $As_2O_3$)

Weak, thirsty, restless patients are best helped by this remedy. Patients who dwindle down to mere skeletons especially when this weakness develops rapidly. Weakness associated with or alternating with restlessness.

*Neuropathy* — The patient complains of burning pains especially in the palms and soles which are better by heat. Neuralgias and multiple neuritis. Also useful in carbuncles and gangrene with cadaverous odor and burning pains which are better by heat. Ulcers on toes and soles with wooden feeling in soles. Dry rough scaly skin. Chilly patients. Dry tongue and mouth with intense thirst but can only drink a little at a time. Inreased quantity of urine with great burning while passing urine. Urine contains albumin.

38

## BORACICUM ACIDUM

### (Boric acid, $H_3BO_3$)

Diabetes with a dry, red, cracked tongue. Though coldness is a marked symptom of this drug, with cold saliva and cold feeling in internal parts like vagina, climacteric flushes are also covered by this drug. Oedema of tissues, especially around the eyes. Frequent urging to urinate.

## BOVISTA
### (Puff-ball)

Especially adapted to old maids with palpitations. Multiple neuritis with numbness and tingling sensation in the affected part. The patients have a frequent desire to urinate sometimes even immediately after urinating. Awkward persons.

## BRYONIA ALBA
### (White bryony, wild hops)

Extreme dryness of the mouth and lips with intense thirst should make one think of Bryonia. Great urging to urinate whenever the intra-abdominal pressure is raised as when lifting something heavy or riding on a rough road. Urine looks brown like beer. Sensation of a stone in the stomach after meals. The region of the liver is sensitive to touch. Constipation with dry hard stools. Hot patient.

## CARBO VEGETABILIS
### (Vegetable charcoal)

Patients with a cold Hippocratic face and cold sweat. Debilitated patients, faint easily; Diabetic Retoacidosis, almost lifeless but the head is hot; the breath is cold, pulse is imperceptible, respiration is oppressed and rapid and the patient desires to be fanned. Septic conditions coupled with a burning sensation. The legs are cold from the knees downward. Gangrene, bed-sores which bleed easily. Indolent ulcers, carbuncles with burning pains.

## CARBOLIC ACID
### (Carbolic acid, Phenol, $C_6H_5OH$)

Carbolic acid suits those patients who are broken down, prostrated. Septic conditions especially in persons who are somnolent, who easily fall asleep. Frequent urination at night more so in old patients. Urine contains albumin and ketones. Intense halitosis with dyspepsia or constipation. Great desire for stimulants.

## CAUSTICUM
### (Tinctura acris sine kali, Potassium Hydrate)

Diabetic neuropathy with paralysis and numbness. Cracking in knees. Stiff muscles with sensation as if the tendons were shortened. Paralysis ameliorated by cold applications even by cold drinks. Emaciation. Cataract.

## CEANOTHUS AMERICANUS
### (New Jersey Tea)

Diabetes in persons with splenic troubles, enlargement and pain in the left side of the abdomen which is worse lying on the left side. Green frothy urine which contains sugar. Diabetes complicated with hypertension.

40

## CEPHALANDRA INDICA
**(Telakucha)**

Dryness of the mouth with great thirst for large quantity of water at a time. Thirsty after passing urine. Loss of appetite. Burning sensation anywhere in the body always better by cold applications. Copious urine followed by exhaustion. Glycosuria.

## CONIUM MACULATUM
**(Poison Hemlock)**

Conium is more often indicated in old persons who present with the following symptoms - exhaustion, fatigue, drowsiness, dryness of skin with itching, dry mouth and tongue, constipation, frequent desire to urinate, cataract, amaurosis, impotence.

## CROTALUS HORRIDUS
**(Rattle-snake)**

This deep acting snake venom should be thought of in septic states, haemorrhages, carbuncles accompanying Diabetes. Boils, carbuncles and ulcers are surrounded by a purplish halo. Right sided affections. All discharges are fetid.

## CUPRUM ARSENICOSUM
**(Arsenite of Copper, Scheele's Green)**

This remedy is eminently suited to a state of dehydration with attendant acidosis. Urine is scanty and contains ketones. Also suited to carbuncles and diabetic gangrene which is always associated with cold sweat. Dark liquid stools with violent abdominal pains.

## CUPRUM METALLICUM
### (Copper, the metal)

Emaciation which progresses slowly but steadily. The patient is very thirsty, has an increased appetite and complains of a sweetish taste in the mouth. Constipation with dry stools in persons who pass large quantities of straw-colored turbid urine.

## FLUORIC ACID
### (Hydrofluoric acid HF)

This remedy is suited to chronic cases which demonstrate a syphilitic taint either in the past or the family history. Complaints of old age or of those who are prematurely old. Alcoholics. Hot patients whose discharges tend to be thin, foul and acrid. This remedy is found more useful when the patient consults you with some full-blown complication of Diabetes like ulcers (which have red edges). Redness of the palms. Diabetes with circulatory troubles of the lower extremities due to atony of the veins and the capillaries.

## GYMNEMA SYLVESTRE
### (Gurmar)

Glycosuria with increased frequency of micturition both day and night. Progressive weakness worse after passing urine. Burning pains in boils and carbuncles. Impotence. Reduces sugar in urine.

## HELLEBORUS NIGER
### (Black Hellebore, Christmas Rose)

The symptomatology of this remedy corresponds to one of the acute medical emergencies - Diabetic

Pre-Coma. The patient is in a low state, he sees and hears imperfectly with generalised muscular weakness. This is most commonly due to hypoglycemia either due to inadequate oral intake or an overdose of insulin or oral hypoglycemic agents. The patient picks at his lips and clothes. There is a constant chewing motion of the jaw. Sighing respiration with slow, small, soft pulse. The patient shrieks and shouts; he cannot be fully aroused. Another characteristic symptom is that the patient greedily swallows water even when unconscious.

## HELONIAS DIOICA
**(Unicorn root)**

Weak, languorous and prostrated persons are best affected by this remedy as also tired backachy females. The patient is always better in all complaints when occupied. Constant aching, burning and tenderness over the kidneys. Urine is profuse and contains albumin, sugar and phosphates. Pruritus vulvae with redness, burning and itching of pudendum. There may be a history of albuminuria during pregnancy.

## IODUM
**(Iodine, the element)**

The symptomatology of Iodum corresponds very strongly to that of Juvenile onset (Type I) Diabetes Mellitus. The patient experiences a progressive loss of weight even though eating well. Debility of recent onset and rapid progress. Iodum acts on glands, first inflaming them and then deranging their function, the patient always feels too hot. This drug is useful in the intercurrent exacerbations of the general state especially by infection, mainly of the respiratory tract, both upper and lower. Patients with a history of nervous-shock, disappointment in love. Copious frequent urination with cuticle on the surface of the urine. Profuse sweating. Constipation better by cold milk.

## IRIS VERSICOLOR
### (Blue Flag)

Diabetes in patients with a tendency to sick headaches which are associated with visual disturbances. Greasy taste in the mouth, with burning of the whole alimentary tract. Profuse clear urine with burning in the urethra after urination. Iris has a marked action on the pancreas.

## KALIUM BROMATUM
### (Potassium bromide, KBr)

Like all the Kali salts, Kali brom. also has a lot of debility. Cases of sensory diabetic neuropathy causing anaesthesia especially of mucous membranes of eyes, throat and of skin. Autonomic neuropathies manifested by impotence though this is usually accompanied by a heightened sexual desire. Broca's aphasia where the patient can repeat whatever he hears but cannot speak by himself. The anaesthesia of the mucous membrane of the throat causes dysphagia for liquids, though solids can be swallowed with relative ease. Fidgety persons. Cerebrovascular accidents in Diabetics. Patients with a tendency to acne, eczema, psoriasis.

## KREOSOTUM
### (Kreosote, a wood tar distillate)

One of the best remedies alongwith Arsenic, Lachesis and Secale for diabetic gangrene with extreme offensiveness and debility. Blackness of the affected part. All discharges are hot, acrid and foul. Tendency to easy caries of teeth, blackening of teeth with weak enamel and spongy bleeding gums. Frequent urination; drinks much but passes little urine at a time. Burning of soles. Violently itching skin eruptions worse in the evening. Periodical haemoptysis in neglected Pulmonary Tuberculosis. Vulvo-vaginitis with corrosive itching within vulva, burning and swelling of labia; violent itching between labia and thighs.

## LACHESIS TRIGONOCEPHALUS
### (Venom of the Surukuku snake)

This is another remedy which is found useful in the treatment of complications rather than the disease itself. Low states of disease — haemorrhage, sepsis, carbuncles, ulcers, bed-sores, cellulitis, gangrene with great prostration. Impotence — strong desire without physical power. Trigeminal neuralgia especially of the left side. Climacteric troubles. Arteriosclerosis. The patient always sleeps into an aggravation. Skin lesions have a bluish, purple appearance and are better by warm application. Alcoholics.

## LACTIC ACID
### (Lactic acid, Milk acid)

Being an acid, this remedy has the characteristic debility of Diabetes. Suitable to anemic ladies, who are pale, who suffer from nausea (which is better by eating) and numerous affections of the breasts. Thirsty, voracious eaters, who pass large quantites of saccharine urine.

## LYCOPODIUM CLAVATUM
### (Club moss, Wolf's claw)

Thin withered persons who suffer from hyperacidity and flatulence (especially in the lower abdomen). Emaciated persons with a withered, shrivelled face. Profuse urine. Easy satiety or canine hunger, the patient may even wake up from sleep at night feeling hungry. Gnawing in the stomach better by drinking hot water. Intellegent persons. Premature greying of hair. Craves sweets. Impotence in old persons with a heightened sexual desire.

## MEDORRHINUM
### (Nosode of Gonorrhoea)

Clarke mentions Diabetes in the clinical symptomatology of this remedy. A family history of gonorrhoea, aggravation of all symptoms from sunrise to sunset, amelioration at the sea-shore, obstinate rheumatism (and sequelae of rheumatism), albuminuria, glandular enlargements, difficulty in mental concentration, impatience are the guiding symptoms to the use of this remedy in Diabetes. The patient cannot speak without crying, which ameliorates. Patient craves salt, sweets, ice, green fruits. Great thirst especially for alcoholic beverages. Itching of the body worse when thinking of it. Neuropathy, burning of the palms and the feet, which though cold to touch, are better when uncovered and fanned.

## MORPHINUM
### (Morphia, an alkaloid of Opium)

A most useful remedy for Diabetic neuropathy. Intensely painful neuralgias better by hot applications. Multiple neuritis. Diabetic Pre-coma and Coma with very dry mouth and great thirst. Difficult swallowing from paralysis of the pharynx; better hot drinks, worse solids. Incessant, deathly nausea with vomitting.

Diarrhoea or constipation with horrible tenesmus. Alternate tachycardia and bradycardia. Diaphragmatic paralysis. Melancholic delirium. Neuralgic pains cause twitching and jerking of limbs.

## MOSCHUS
### (Secretion of the preputial follicles of the Musk Deer)

Diabetes Mellitus in hysterical women. Selfish, obstinate, much-pampered persons who will resort to anything to get their way. Persons with a tendency to easy fainting. Coldness in general or of single parts is an unfailing guide to this remedy. Impotence. Profuse watery urine which is normal during the day but dark and offensive at night.

## NATRUM MURIATICUM
### (Sodium Chloride, Common Salt, NaCL)

This remedy must be chosen essentially as a constitutional prescription. Thin, thirsty, HOT, emaciated, poorly nourished persons. Tearfulness and weeping tendency as a concomittant of all complaints. Emaciation though eating well. Tendency to take cold. Complaints after Malaria, Quinine, too much Salt, Loss of Fluids, Fright, Grief, Disappointment. Patient dwells on past disagreeable events. Fear or dreams of robbers. Polyuria with thirst for large quantities of water. Has to wait a long time to pass urine especially in the presence of others. Numbness and tingling of the lower extremities. Dry mucous membrances. Great weakness and weariness.

## NATRUM SULPHURICUM
### (Sodium Sulphate, Glauber's Salt, $Na_2SO_4$)

Diabetes in patients with a Sycotic taint. Useful in

patients with a hydrogenoid constitution who pass profuse urine and suffer from a lot of flatulence. Itching of skin worse while undressing. Obese patients suffering from rheumatism. Consequences of living in damp houses, basements etc. Sycotic excrescences.

## NITRIC ACID
### (Nitric acid, $HNO_3$)

Diabetic ulcers with zigzag, ragged edges, profuse granulation and bleeding easily on touch. Ulcers with splinter-like pains. Cases with a sycotic and syphilitic background. Offensive urine smelling like horses' urine. Urine cold on passing.

## NUX VOMICA
### (Strychnos Nur Vomica, Poison Nut)

Suited to persons who suffer from ill-effects of irregularity of food and sleep. Chilly patients debilitated by business tensions and debauches. Irritable, sullen, fault-finding persons addicted to smoking, alcohol and stimulants. Constipation with frequent ineffectual urge to pass stool. Frequent desire to urinate. Desire for stimulants.

## OPIUM
### (Papaver Somniferum, Poppy)

Diabetic coma. Heavy, stupid sleep with stertorous breathing and sweaty skin. Pupils constricted. Complete loss of consciousness. Delirious talking with eyes wide open. Breathing stops on going to sleep, must be shaken to start it again. Obstinate constipation, no urge; round hard black ball-like stools. Pulse full and slow. Hot sweat.

## PHOSPHORICUM ACIDUM
### (Phosphoric acid, $H_3PO_4$)

Diabetes Mellitus in nervous patients. Profuse milky urine loaded with sugar and phosphates. Bad effects of Grief, Worry, Anxiety. Indifferent, apathetic and debilitated.Loss of appetite with extreme thirst. Bruised feeling in the muscles. Somnolence. Profuse sweat. Young people who grow rapidly and are overtaxed mentally and physically. Premature greying and falling of hair. Impotence. Ulcers on the skin are painless and exude a very offensive pus. Formication in various parts. Neuralgia after ambutation of stump. Amblyopia.

## PHOSPHORUS
### (Phosphorus, the element. P)

Eminently suited to patients with a tubercular history either in the past or in the family. Young persons of a nervous temperament who grow rapidly and are inclined to stoop. Gradually increasing debility. Very sensitive to external impressions - sound, odor, light, touch, electrical changes, thunderstorms. Pain and burning in spots. Falling out of hair in large bunches. Thirst for very cold water, to the extent that patients crave ice-cubes, which is vomitted out as soon as it gets warm in the stomach. Turbid brown urine. Impotence with strong desire. Sterility with nymphomania. Cataract, amblyopia, diplopia, lesions of the retina and the optic nerve.

## PICRICUM ACIDUM
### (Picric acid, C6H2(NO2)30H)

Weakness, heavy tired feeling in the body and mind. Easy prostration. Pins and needles sensation in the whole body. Ammoniacal urine which dribbles. Albuminuria with granular and hyaline casts. Pruritus vulvae.

## PLUMBUM METALLICUM
### (Lead, the element Pb)

Motor and sensory neuritis. Partial anaesthesia with paralysis chiefly of the extensor muscles. Paralysis of single muscles; paralysis from overexertion of the extensor muscles in piano players. Wrist drop. Neuralgic pains better by pressure. Arteriosclerosis and hypertension. Albuminuria. Constipation with hard black ball-like stools. Bedsores. Dry burning ulcers. Small wounds easily inflamed and suppurate.

## SANICULA AQUA
### (A mineral spring water of Ottawa, Ill., U.S.A.)

Cachexia, ravenous appetite, increased thirst and profuse urination point to the usefulness of this drug in the treatment of Diabetes Mellitus. Weakness, emaciation, with dirty, greasy, ill-nourished skin which itches intolerably. Cold clammy hands and feet with foul sweat. Stubborn constipation, no desire for days; also diarrhoea with green stools having odor of rotten cheese. Frequent urge to pass urine. Great effort needed to retain urine, at times impossible, yet if desire is resisted, the urging ceases.

## SECALE CORNUTUM
### (Ergot of Rye)

One of the most important remedies for diabetic gangrene. Numbness and icy-coldness of the extremities. Blue colour of the skin. Dry gangrene developing slowly. Burning pains as if sparks of fire were falling on the skin better by cold application, patient wants the part uncovered though it is cold to the touch. Formication under the skin. Great aversion to heat and covering. Large ecchymoses. Gangrene of the genitalia. The extreme offensiveness of Arsenic, Kreosote and Lachesis is not found in this drug.

## SEPIA
### (Inky juice of the Cuttle-fish)

Persons of both the sexes, of nervous and delicate constitution who are disposed to sexual excitement or worn out by sexual excesses. Weak, pot-bellied persons with a yellow complexion. Complaints start at or are worse at menopause. Characteristic ball-like sensation internally. Great prostration though the patient is generally better by physical exertion. Empty all gone sensation in the stomach not better by eating. Profuse offensive sweating. Involuntary urination on coughing or sneezing. Extremities cold even in a warm room.

## SILICEA
### (Silicea terra, Pure flint, Silicon dioxide, $SiO_2$)

Neurasthenia due to imperfect assimilation and defective nutrition. Suppurative proceses, sinuses, abscesses, fistulae, felons. Slow incomplete inflammation followed by induration. Want of moral and physical grit. Extremely CHILLY patient. Thirsty. Intolerance of alcohol. Sweaty and icy-cold feet; offensive foot sweat. Bad effects of suppressed foot sweat. Every little injury suppurates; pus is offensive. Frequent urging to pass urine with tenesmus.

## SULPHUR
### (Sulphur the element, S)

Frequent urge to pass urine. Urgency, must hurry, sudden call to urinate. Passes great quantities of colorless urine. Thirsty patient. Burning pains, ebulitions of heat, dislike of water and washing. Dirty unhealthy skin. Redness of the orifices. Empty all gone, sinking feeling in the epigastrium at about 11 a.m. Early morning diarrhoea.

## SYZYGIUM JAMBOLANUM
### (Kala Jaam, Jambul)

Diabetes Mellitus with intense thirst, polyuria and dry mouth. Diabetic ulcers, both acute as well as chronic. Prickly heat in the upper part of the body. Has a wonderful effect on the blood sugar, lowers it almost immediately, causing glycosuria. (Syzygium has been shown to decrease glycosuria caused by Phloridzin, but Phloridzin itself causes only renal glycosuria and has no effect on blood sugar).

## TARENTULA CUBENSIS
### (Cuban Spider)

Very few direct references to the use of Tarentula in Diabetes are found in our literature. Margaret Tyler quotes Hering and I quote her 'Diabetes Mellitus with craving for raw articles'. Other symptoms are polyuria with numbness of the legs. Carbuncles, deep abscesses etc. which are surrounded by purplish skin. Persons easily affected by seeing others in trouble and who are disgusted by meat.

52

## THUJA OCCIDENTALIS
### (Arbor Vitae, Tree of Life)

.Hahnemann's king of the anti-sycotic remedies. Diabetes in persons who have a past history of gonorrhoea and/or vaccination. Persons who have fixed ideas and identity crises. Hydrogenoid constitution of Grauvogl. Tearing pains in the joints and the muscles worse in damp, humid atmosphere, at rest and better in dry weather. Rapid exhaustion and emaciation. Chilly patients. Fig warts and condylomata. Inveterate tea drinkers who suffer from it's bad effects. Flat ulcers with a bluish floor.

## URANIUM NITRICUM
### (Uranium Nitrate, $UO_2NO_3$ $6H_2O$)

Great emaciation, debility with tendency to ascites and general dropsy. Excessive thirst, nausea and vomitting. Ravenous appetite yet the patient is greatly emaciated. Polyuria, glycosuria usually associated with hypertension. Dryness of the mouth and the skin. The principle remedy when Diabetes originates in dyspepsia or is due to disorders of assimilation. Associated gastric or duodenal ulcers.

## *RARE REMEDIEIS*

Adrenalin

Alumina

Ammonium Aceticum

Anthrokokali

Aristolochia Milhomens

Arnica Montana

Arsenicum Bromatum

Asclepias Vincetoxicum

Asparagus

Belladonna

Calcarea Phosphoricum

Carlsbad

Chimaphila Umbellata

Chloralum

Coca

Codeinum

Colchicum
Crataegus
Curare
Ferrum Iodatum
Ferrum Muriaticum
Ficus Indica
Glycerinum
Hydrangea
Insulin
Kali Aceticum
Kissingen
Lac Vaccinum
Lac Vaccinum Defloratum
Lecithin
Lycopersicum
Lycopus
Magnesium Sulph

Manganum
Natrum Phos
Oxygenium
Pancreatinum
Phaseolus
Plantago
Phloridzin
Podophyllum
Quinin Mur
Rhus Aromatica
Saccharum Lactis
Saccharum Officinale
Strychnin Ars
Taraxacum
Thyroidinum
Urea
Vanadium

## ADRENALIN
### (Extract of the Supra-renal glands, a Sarcode)

Clarke mentions it as having cured the following symtoms : Loss of strength, wasting, bronzing of the skin. Thus, Adrenalin may be found useful in' Bronzed Diabeates' which is a variety of Diabetes secondary to Haemochromatosis.

## ALUMINA
### (Aluminium Oxide, $Al_2O_3$, $3H_2O$)

Alumina has been very highly recommended by Rai Bahadur Bishamber Das as almost specific for Diabetic Coma, but he does not mention any characteristic indication.

# AMMONIUM ACETICUM
## (Ammonium acetate, $C_2H_3O_2NH_4$)

Profuse saccharine urine with profuse sweat. "Bathed in Sweat" Warmth in the abdomen; in the skin.

# ANTHROKOKALI
## (Anthracite coal dissolved in boiling caustic potash)

Dryness of mouth, throat with internal heat extending to the stomach. Chronic cracks of the nostrils. Great thirst with abundant flow of urine. Itching of the skin worse in the night. Pustular eruptions.

# ARISTOLOCHIA MILHOMENS
## (Brazillian snake-root)

Copius urine with intense thrist, Bitter taste in the mouth, pasty mouth. Concomittant - Flatulence; Pricking, lacinating pains in various parts; pains taking away the breath.

# ARNICA MONTANA
## (Leopard's bane)

Dryness of the mouth with increased thirst and frequent desire to urinate with copius urine. Arnica is mentioned as being useful in cases where diabetes starts after a blow on the liver.

# ARSENICUM BROMATUM
## (Bromide of arsenic, $AsBr_3$)

Diabetes Mellitus with great thirst and constipation, Loss of weight and tendency to cutaneous eruptions like acne, furuncles, anthrax.

## ASCLEPIAS VINCETOXICUM
### (Swallow-wart)

Diabetes Mellitus with dropsy, great thirst and profuse urine. Insatiable hunger. Vomiting and purging.

## ASPARAGUS
### (Asparagus officinalis)

Sensation of fullness of the abdomen with flatulence and eructations. Increased thirst with frequent desire to pass abundant straw-coloured urine. Sensation as if there was more urine to pass.

## BELLADONNA
### (Atropa Belladonna, Deadly Nightshade)

It is mentioned as being indicated in Diabetes after a head injury. (This is of cource not true Diabetes but is a stress induced phenomenon due to release of adrenal hormones.)

## CALCAREA PHOSPHORICUM
### (Phosphate of Lime, $Ca_3(PO_4)_2$)

Diabetes with lung complications, of great service not only to the lungs but also in diminishing the quantity of urine and lowering its specific gravity. Chronic cough, profuse sweats.

## CARLSBAD
### (Waters of the Sprudel and Muhlbrunnen Springs)

Diabetes with extreme prostration; so weak that the patient trembles, speech is low. Constipation due to weak action of the bowels. Profuse urine. All the symptoms are better in open air and by movement.

## CHIMAPHILA UMBELLATA
### (Pipsissewa, Prince's pine)

May be found to be of use in cases with a sycotic taint who develop diabetic nephropathy. Sugar in the urine. Hypertrophy of the prostate. Urine contains a mucopurulent deposit.

## CHLORALUM
### (Chloral hydrate, $C_2HCl_3O$ $H_2O$)

Diabetes mellitus with sleeplessness and an over-worked or fagged brain. Profuse urination.

## COCA
### (Erthoxylon coca)

Diabetes Mellitus with impotence.

## CODEINUM
### (An Alkaloid of Opium, $C_{18}H_{21}NO_3$)

Diabetes with itching and sensation of warmth of the skin. Numbness of parts. Glycosuria.

## COLCHICUM AUTUMNALE
### (Meadow Saffron)

Diabetes complicated by gouty symptoms. The patient is prostrated and complains of internal cold-ness. The patient is thirsty and craves effervescent alcoholic drinks. Nausea caused by the mere sight or smell of food. The urine contains albumin and sugar.

## CRATAEGUS OXYACANTHA
### (Hawthorn)

Phatak mentions this remedy for Diabetes in children but gives no further pointers to its use.

## CURARE
### (An arrow poison used by South American Indians)

Scrophulus persons. Fetid discharges. Emaciation, glycosuria, dry mouth, great thirst and copious urine. Numbness and tingling of the extremities. Diabetic coma with paralysis of the respiratory muscles and diminished reflexes.

## FERRUM IODATUM
### (Iodide of iron, $FeI_2$)

Sweet-smelling urine. Feels as if she had eaten too much, a sort of upward pressure. Stuffed feeling in the abdomen as if she could not lean forwards. Constipation. Glandular enlargements. Rectal concomitants. Dryness of mouth and throat with great thirst. Greasy acrid eructations. Frequent profuse urine. Albuminuria.

## FERRUM MURIATICUM
### (Ferrous Chloride, $FeCl_2$ $4H_2O$)

Diabetes with an insipid flat taste in the mouth and dry mouth. Tongue is coated. Haematuria. Unquenchable thirst. Craving for acids.

## FICUS INDICA
### (Ficus Bengalensis, Banyan tree)

Diabetes with burning pain in the urethra during micturition and haematuria.

## GLYCERINUM
### (Pure glycerine)

Clarke quotes Cooper as saying that is the thirsti-est plant known and has used it in cases of Diabetes presenting with great thirst and abdominal symp-toms. Profuse urine with white amorphous deposit.

## INSULIN
### (A secretion of the pancreas, a sarcode)

Its use has been suggested in cases with persis-tent skin irritation, boils and ulceration with polyuria. It is said to be of use in carbuncles.

## KALI ACETICUM
### (Potassium acetate, $KC_2H_3O_2$)

Diabetes with diarrhoea, dropsy and profuse al-kaline urine.

## KISSINGEN
### (Springs of Kissingen in Bavaria)

Trembling of the whole body, weariness. Pulsation of the entire body. Tearful disposition - "If he only looks at someone he must weep." Muscae volitantes. Tinnitus.

## LAC VACCINUM
### (Cow's milk)

Frequent discharge of profuse clear urine, no sediment; this coupled with great thirst points to its use in Diabetes. Great physical prostration. Symp-toms appear on both sides simultaneously. Vertigo more on closing the eyes. Occipital headache. Obstinate constipation.

## LAC VACCINUM DEFLORATUM
### (Skimmed cow's milk)

Frequent and profuse urination which may be involuntary especially while walking in cold air, while riding or when hurrying to catch a bus or train. Diabetic bladder - lack of sensation when the bladder is full. Chilly patient. Obstinate constipation, sick headaches and car sickness.

## LECITHIN
### (A phospholipid extracted from the yolk of egg and animal brains.)

It is said to improve the nutrition and reduce weakness and hence is a useful adjunct to therapy. Impotence. Glycosuria.

## LYCOPERSICUM ESCULENTUM
### (Solanum lycopersicum, Tomato)

Diabetes with rheumatic pains worse by motion and especially affecting the right deltoid. Headche better by warm applications. Contracted pupils. Coryza on going outdoors.

## LYCOPUS VIRGINICUS
### (Bungle-weed)

Intense thirst, profuse urine. Diabetes with heart complaints. Haemoptysis from valvular heart defects. Diabetes with Thyroid disease, exophthalmos.

## MAGNESIUM SULPHURICUM
### (Epsom salts, $MgSO_4$ $7H_2O$)

All complaints — diarrhoea, chill etc. — accompanied by great thirst. Copious stools. Great lassitude with soreness of the whole body. Tendency to boils. Nausea with coldness in the stomach. Digust for meat.

## MANGANUM
### (Manganum aceticum, $Mn(C_2H_3O_2)_2$ $4H_2O$)

Phatak, in his repertory, mentions only Manganum under the rubric - Itching, Diabetes in. Also useful for malignant ulcers with blue borders following slight injury.

## NATRUM PHOSPHORICUM
### (Phospate of soda, $Na_2HPO_4$ $12H_2O$)

Tyler points to its use in Diabetes but gives no special indications other than a thick, moist, creamy or golden -yellow coated tongue, sour eructations, sour vomiting and hyperacidity. Phatak says that it is useful for Diabetes with successive boils.

## OXYGENIUM
### (Oxygen the element, O)

Clarke mentions the cure of a case of Diabetes with large doses of Oxygenium but does not elaborate further.

## PANCREATIN
### (Extract of Pancreatic glands of Ox or Sheep)

An organ remedy; has been used with success in conditions due to disease or faulty action of the Pancreas, i.e. secondary Diabetes.

## PHASEOLUS NANUS
**(Dwarf-bean)**

Diabetes with palpitations and a weak pulse. Dropsical effusion into the pleural or pericardial cavities.

## PLANTAGO MAJOR
**(Plantain)**

Halitosis, sinking and weight in the stomach with flatulence, diarrhoea and hearty appetite. Copious urine with increased nocturnal frequency and increased thirst. Tingling in urethra and itching in the meatus. Inflammatory conditions of skin and cellular tissue. Itching parts burn after scratching.

## PHLORIDZIN
**(A glucoside isolated form the root of apple and other friut trees.)**

Diabetes with fatty degeneration of the liver. Causes renal glycosuria, has no effect on blood sugar.

## PODOPHYLLUM PELTATUM
**(May apple)**

Useful in Diabetes of pregnancy with large, moist, coated tongue. Loss of taste. Thirst for large quantity of cold water. The classical diarrhoea may or may not be present. Prolapse of rectum.

## QUININ MURIATICUM
**(Quinine Hydrochloride)**

Removes sugar from the urine.

## RHUS AROMATICA
### (Fragrant Sumach)

Diabetes with weakness; slightest work tires her. Backache. Appetite alternately ravenous and diminished.

## SACCHARUM LACTIS
### (Lactose)

Diabetes with "cold Pains". Neuralgias worse least breath of air, slighest touch. Pains are icy cold as if produced by extremely fine ice-cold needles. Hungry all the time. Great thirst for large quantities of cold water.

## SACCHARUM OFFICINALE
### (Sugar, $C_{12}H_{22}O_{11}$)

Cataract, amblyopia and opacity of the cornea, all known complications of Diabetes, have been reported cured by the use of potentised Sac. off.

## STRYCHNINUM ARSENICOSUM
### (Arsenite of Strychnin an alkaloid of Nux Vomice)

Prostration, fatty degenration with hypertrophy of the heart. Scanty urine loaded with sugar. Complaints of old age. Chronic diarrhoea.

## TARAXACUM
### (Dandelion)

Diabetes with frequent profuse urination in persons with gastric headaches, bilious complaints, jaundice and the characteristic mapped tongue.

## THYROIDINUM
### (Thyroid gland of the sheep or calf, A sarcode)

Great thirst for cold water. Increased flow of urine which smells of violets. Easy fatigue, fainting fits. Rapid emaciation. Decided craving for large quantities of sugar. Delayed union of fractutes. palpitations. Premature greying of hair.

## UREA PURA
### (Urea, $CO(NH_2)_2$)

It is mentioned as useful in Diabetes and uremia. Constant urging to urinate with albuminaria.

## VANADIUM
### (Vanadium, the metal)

Its action as an oxygen carrier and catalyst points to its use in wasting diseases in general. Acts as a tonic to the digestive function. Atherosclerosis.

# 11.
# REFERENCES IN THE REPERTORY

Diabetes Mellitus, essentially being a nosological diagnosis, is not always directly represented in the repertories. For example, Kent's repertory does not give a direct rubric for diabetes though the condition is amply covered by rubrics like Urine copious, Urine sugar, Urine albuminous, Urine specific gravity increased etc. Thirst increased, Extremities pain Burning (neuropathy), Carbuncles are other rubrics which can be utilised. Symptoms of Diabetes as well as its complications are well covered in Kent's repertory.

Similarly, in the repertories of Boger, Lippe and Knerr the representation is essentially in the chapter of Urine though Knerr gives a rubric 'Urine, Diabetes'.

The repertories of Boericke and Phatak alongwith the works of Homoeopathic therapeutics by Lilienthal, Dewey, Hughes and Bishamber Das mention Diabetes directly.

# 12.
# DIETETICS

In this chapter we will attempt to look at the broad outline of dietetics and nutrition in a diabetic patient. A diabetic has essentially the same need of nutrients as a normal person, but his ability to metabolise these nutrients efficiently and rapidly is hampered to a greater or lesser extent. This necessitates a modification in the diabetic's dietary intake. Besides, appropriate dietary modification may even do away with the need for active medical management.

Let us first look at caloric requirement of normal individuals:

## Table no. - 1

Normal Caloric Requirement according to age.

| Group | | | Calories |
|---|---|---|---|
| Children | 1 to 3 | years | 1200 |
| | 4 to 6 | years | 1500 |
| | 7 to 9 | years | 1800 |
| | 10 to 12 | years | 2100 |
| Adolescents | | | 2300 to 3000 |
| Men | Sedentary work | | 2400 |
| | Moderate work | | 2800 |
| | Heavy work | | 3900 |
| Women | Sedentary work | | 1900 |
| | Moderate work | | 2200 |
| | Heavy work | | 3000 |
| Pregnancy | | | Normal + 300 to 400 |
| Lactation | | | Normal + 600 to 700 |

Now let us briefly cast a glance over the different constituents of a balanced diet.

## CARBOHYDRATES

These are ready sources of energy for the human body. They can be broadly differentiated into (i) Simple sugars like sugar, honey etc. and (ii) Complex starches like rice, cereal, flour etc. Cereals, flours, dairy products, fruits and vegetables are good sources of carbohydrate. The normal daily requirement of carbohydrate is about 4 to 6 gm/kg body weight. A minimum of 100 gms of carbohydrate daily is essential to prevent excess fat breakdown and ketosis. Concentrated carbohydrates like sugar and sweets are rapidly absorbed and hence raise blood glucose levels rapidly. Complex carbohydrates (starches) are preferable because they are absorbed slowly and hence cause lesser fluctuations in blood glucose levels.

## PROTEINS

Proteins are complex compounds required by the body for the maintenance, growth and repair of the tissues. Proteins are formed of basic building blocks called Amino acids which may be either an essential or non-essential amino-acid. Milk, Milk Products, eggs, meat and nuts are rich in proteins. Fruits, vegetables, cereals and pulses have a low to moderate protein content. Usually adults require 55 to 75 gms of proteins daily. This requirement rises during growth, pregnancy and lactation. Proteins help to sustain blood glucose levels in the period between meals and hence guard against hypoglycaemia.

## FATS

Fats or Lipids are a very rich source of calories. Fats containing a large percentage of polyunsaturated fatty acids are to be preferred. The daily intake of fat should be such that it supplise approximately 20 per cent of the total calories. The type of fats in the diet is important. Diabetic vasculopathy is a known complication and hence diabetic diets should be low in saturated fats and cholesterol.

## VITAMINS AND MINERALS

The total daily requirement of vitamins and minerals of a diabetic is in no way different from that of a normal person.

## FIBRE

Fibre is a type of carbohydrate that is not digested in the digestive tract of humans. It contributes little to the nutritive value but provides roughage in the diet. Vegetables, fruits, whole grain and bran are rich sources of fibre. Fibre delays carbohydrate absorption and slows down the post-prandial rise of blood glucose. Moderate amounts of fibre helps lower serum cholesterol and may promote weight loss.

## THE EXCHAGE SYSTEM

This is based on the fact that all the food items can be grouped into seven basic types. Articles under the same heading can be interchanged safely with each other as they have almost identical carbohydrate, protein and fat content. However they are not usually interchang able with articles under other groups.

The basic food groups and their contents are given on the following page :-

| Food | | Quantity = 1 exchange | Calories | Carbohydrate gms | Proteins gms | Fats gms |
|---|---|---|---|---|---|---|
| Milk | — Standard | 250 ml | 170 | 12 | 8 | 10 |
| | — Skim | 250 ml | 80 | 12 | 8 | 0 |
| Vegetables | Group A | | | NEGLIGIBLE | | |
| | Group B | 150 gm | 40 | 7 | 2 | 0 |
| Fruit | | (see) | 40 | 10 | 0 | |
| Cereals | | 20 gm | 70 | 15 | 2 | 0 |
| Meat | — Lean | 30 gm | 55 | 0 | 7 | 3 |
| | — Medium fat | 30 gm | 75 | 0 | 7 | 5 |
| | — High fat | 30 gm | 100 | 0 | 7 | 8 |
| Fat | | 5 gm | 45 | 0 | 0 | 5 |
| Pulses | | 20 gm | 70 | 13 | 4 | 0 |

## *Vegetable Group A*

These can be taken in unrestricted amounts.
- Bitter gourd (Karela)
- Cabbage (gobi)
- Capsicum (chillies)
- Cauliflower (phool gobi)
- Cluster beans (gover)
- Cucumbers
- Egg plant (brinjal, baigan)
- Green leafy vegetables
- Lady finger
- Radish (mula)
- Tomatoes

## *Vegetable Group B*

**1 exchange = 150 gms**
- Beetroot
- Doodhi
- Carrot
- French beans
- Green peas
- Onion
- Pumpkin (Kaddu)

# FRUITS

**1 exchange equals**

| | | | |
|---|---|---|---|
| Apple | 1 small | 80 | gms |
| Banana | 1/2 small | 50 | gms |
| Figs | 2 | 50 | gms |
| Grapes | 12 | 75 | gms |
| Mango | 1/2 small | 70 | gms |
| Orange | 1 small | 100 | gms |
| Papaya | 1/2 | 100 | gms |

| Peach | 1 | 100 gms |
| Pear | 1 | 100 gms |
| Pineapple | 1/2 cup | 80 gms |
| Watermelon | 1 cup | 175 gms |

## CEREAL GROUP

### 1 exchange =

| Flour from wheat, jowar or Bajra | 20 gms |
| Rice, Khichdi, Macaroni | 100 gms |
| Bread (1 slice) | 25 gms |

## PULSES GROUP

### 1 exchange =

Channa, Channa dal, Udad, Vaal, Moong, Musoor, any other dal 100 gms

## MEAT GROUP

### 1 exchange = 30 gms

| i) | Lean meat | — Fish |
| | | — Chicken |
| | | — Cottage Cheese (from skimmed milk) |
| ii) | Medium fat Meat | — Ham, Beef (boiled) |
| | | — Brain, Liver, Kidney |
| | | — Cottage Cheese (from whole milk) |
| | | — Egg |
| iii) | High Fat Meat | — Corned beef |
| | | — Cold cuts |
| | | — Cheddar cheese |
| | | — Duck |

## FAT GROUP

### 1 exchange =

Butter, oil, Ghee 5 gms (1 teaspoon)
Groundnuts, Cashew nuts, Almonds 10 gms (5-6 small nuts)

## SIMPLE GUIDELINES FOR A DIABETIC DIET
### Foods to avoid.

Sugar, Glucose.
Cakes, Sweet biscuits
Jam, Marmalade, Chocolate spread.
Honey
Cream, soups and sauces.
Fried food
Fat meat, fat beef
Meat or fish pate
Sausages
Mayonaise, salad dressing.
Sweets, Chocolates, Candy.
Sweetened fruits, desserts
Cream Cheese.
Sweentened drinks, condensed milk.

### Foods to eat in moderation

White bread
Plain unsweetened biscuits
Polished rice
Fish
Eggs
Cornflour
Whole milk, milk drinks (unsweetened)
Unsweetened fruit juices
Dry fruits, nuts
Plain ice cream, pudding Cereals

Yoghurt
Cheese

## Foods to eat in plenty

Wholemeal bread
wholemeal biscuits
wholemeal breakfast cereeals
Sugar-free drinks
Sugar-free sweeteners
Skimmed milk
Fresh fruits
All vegetables

# GUIDELINES FOR A LOW CHOLESTEROL DIET

Factors besides advancing age belived to hasten the hardening of the arteries (atherosolerosis) are Diabetes Mellitus, High Blood Pressure, Cigarette smoking, Overeating and Alcohol intake to name but a few. In view of this, it is desirable for a Diabetic to also regulate the amount of Cholesterol in his diet. The aim of dietary therapy is to reduce and maintain at normal levels the patient's serum cholesterol while supplying a nutritionally complete diet. These measures include:

● Reduction of total fat.
● Reduction of cholesterol.
● Reduction of saturated fat (animal origin)
● Increased intake of unsaturated fat (vegetable origin)

## Foods to AVOID

Coconut oil, Sunflower,
Meat and Bacon fat
Hydrogenated vege-
table oils

## Foods to PREFER

Peanut or corn oil
Lean cuts of meat, bacon.
Unsaturated vegetable oils.

| | |
|---|---|
| Whole Milk. | Skimmed Milk |
| Ice cream. | Low fat ice cream. |
| Egg yolk, | Egg white. |
| Butter, Cheese. | Margarine, low-fat cheese. |
| Whole milk yoghurt. | Low-fat or non-fat yoghurt. |
| Fried foods. | Broiled foods. |
| Cakes, Pastries, Pies. | Cookies (home-made with unsaturated oils and egg white.) |

# 13.
# BIBLIOGRAPHY

1)  Ahmad S.- A Short Repertory to the Indian Drugs.

2)  Allen J.H. - The Chronic Miasms.

3)  Anshutz E. P.- New, Old and Forgotten Remedies.

4)  Bernoville F.- Diabetes Mellitus

5)  Boericke W.-  Pocket Manual of Homcepathic Mateira Medica.

6)  Boericke W. & Dewey W. - The Twelve Tissue Remedies.

7)  Boger C.M. - Boenninghausen's Characteristics and Repertory.

8)  Clarke J.H. - Clinical Reperotory

9)  Clarke J.H.- Dictionary of Practical Materia Medica

10) Das B. - Select Your Remedy.

11) Dewey W. - Practical Homoepathic Therapeutics.

12) Farrington E.A. - Clinical Materia Medica.

13) Ghose S.C. - Drugs of Hindoosthan

14) Hering C. -The Guiding Symptons of our Materia Medica.

15) Hughes R. - Principles and Practice of Homeopathy.

16) Kent J.T.- Repertory of the Homoepathic Materia Medica

17) Knerr C.B. - Repertory of Hering's Guiding Symptoms.

18) Lilienthal S. - Homoeopathic Therapeutics.

19) Mathur K.N. - Diabetes Mellitus, Its Diagonsis and Treatment.

20) Morgan W. - Diabetes Mellitus

21) Phatak S.R. - Materia Medica of Homoeopathic Remedies.

22) Phatak S.R.- A concise Repertory of Homoeopathic Medicines.

23) Ruddock E.H. - Homoeopathic Vade Mecum.

24) Tyler M.L. - Homoeopathic Drug Pictures.